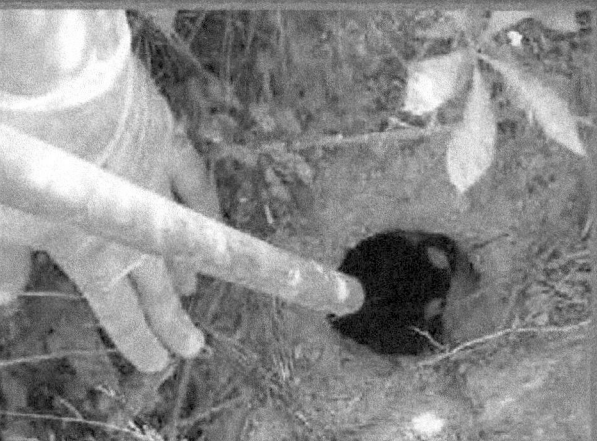
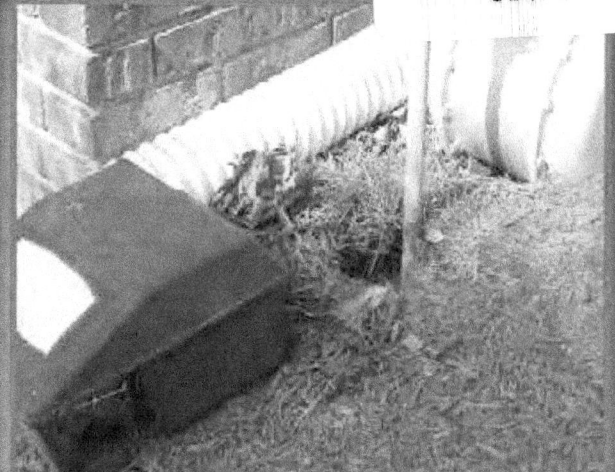
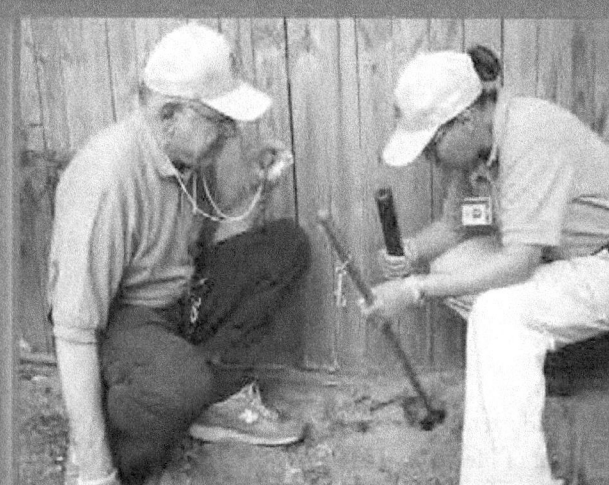
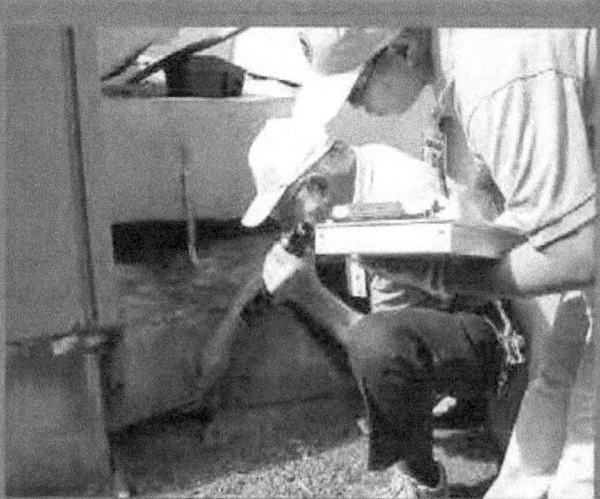

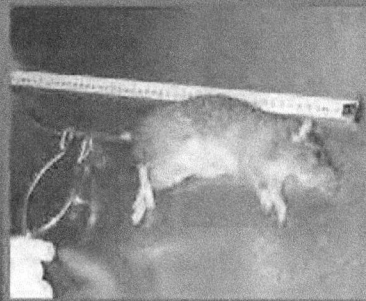

Centers for Disease Control and Prevention

Integrated Pest Management:
Conducting Urban Rodent Surveys

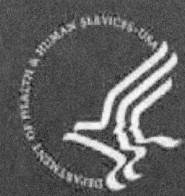

Suggested citation: Centers for Disease Control and Prevention. Integrated pest management: conducting urban rodent surveys. Atlanta: US Department of Health and Human Services; 2006.

Contents

This manual is for classroom use and for field training of program managers, environmental health practitioners, inspectors, outreach workers, and others who work in community-based rodent integrated pest management programs. The manual is also a reference for survey techniques and for the preparation of reports and maps.

Introduction

For centuries, people have recognized that rats and mice are not only a nuisance but are a public health problem. Rats and mice damage and contaminate food, damage structures, and carry diseases that threaten health and quality of life, and they can cause injury and death. This manual describes techniques to help us protect ourselves from these disease vectors by gathering information (surveillance) about infestations and about the causative conditions of infestation. Accurate recordkeeping by public health officials provides the information needed to manage rodent and other pest problems.

Urban rodent surveys of exterior areas are the primary means for obtaining information on rodent infestations and on premises with environmental health deficiencies that support commensal rodent populations in housing and on premisess. Survey areas should include residential, commercial, and civic buildings; vacant lots; and public areas. The rodent species primarily targeted in surveys are the Norway rat (*Rattus norvegicus*), roof rat (*Rattus rattus*), and house mouse (*Mus musculus*).

Urban rodent surveys, as well as surveys for other pests, fulfill an essential surveillance requirement for every integrated pest management (IPM) program, which is the need for detailed information about conditions in a defined community. IPM is a long-term, effective, and holistic approach to managing pests of all kinds by carefully combining various interventions (e.g., education, code enforcement, rodent proofing, poisoning) in ways that minimize environmental hazards and deficiencies that affect people's health.

The focus of this manual is on how to conduct a survey, although the other IPM components are covered briefly to establish their link to the survey. This manual is for classroom use and for the field training of program managers, environmental health practitioners, outreach workers, inspectors, and others who work in community-based rodent IPM programs.

This manual is also a reference on survey techniques and on the preparation of reports and maps.

IPM Basics

Definition and Philosophy

IPM requires a shift from the typical pest control efforts that often emphasize poisoning and trapping. With IPM, pests and disease vectors are managed by managing the environment. For IPM to succeed, the behavior and ecology of the target pest, the environment in which the pest is active, and the periodic changes that occur in the environment (including the people who share the environment) must be taken into account. In addition, the safety of the people, the environment, and the nontarget animals such as pets, birds, and livestock must be considered.

IPM is a decision-making process in which all interventions are focused on a pest problem and on the goal of providing the safest and most effective, economical, and sustained remedy. IPM is a comprehensive systems approach.

IPM is based on and should adhere to the sound biologic principles of population dynamics—the study of birth rates, mortality rates, and movement rates. An understanding of population dynamics is important because any successful strategy for the management of rodent populations depends on that understanding and on conducting appropriate interventions based on IPM principles. A 1976 CDC publication on urban rat control states that

> *"political mechanisms must be able to administer the control procedures that are dictated by the principles [of population dynamics]. ...A corollary of the strategy of working with principles is that research should not continue in clear violation of population principles in expectation that a politically acceptable solution will be found."*

Program and political support are essential in obtaining the necessary resources for an IPM program that takes into account the complex interplay of rodents, people, and environmental factors. The overall goals of IPM are to reduce or eliminate human encounters with pests and disease vectors and to reduce pesticide exposure.

Program Components

The four key components of an IPM program are survey, tolerance limit, intervention, and evaluation. If a key component is omitted, success in managing or eliminating pests is reduced.

Surveys (inspection and monitoring): A measure of the magnitude of the pest problem and its environmental causes. Survey results determine the need for a rodent IPM program and the direction the program must take to manage the rodent problem. An urban rodent survey has four distinct phases:

1. premises inspection (comprehensive or sample) of defined areas (e.g., groups of blocks) to record infestations and their causative conditions;

2. preparation of maps, graphs, and tables to summarize survey results (may include photographs of field observations);

3. preparation of a report that includes an analysis of block and premises data, and premises prevalence rates for infestation and its causative conditions; and

4. recommendations to resolve the rodent infestation problem.

Surveys are especially useful in the development of educational interventions directed to the public (e.g., Web sites, television and radio programs, videos, newspaper articles, brochures, posters, exhibits).

Tolerance limit (action threshold): The level at which a pest causes sufficient damage to warrant public health attention and intervention. Real or perceived damage can be aesthetic and can have economic, psychologic, and medical consequences. In 1972, CDC established tolerance limits for rodent infestation, exposed garbage, and improperly stored refuse. Details of these and other survey-based criteria are discussed later in this manual. The survey establishes the baseline on rodent infestation and on the causative conditions that support the infestation. The goal is to reduce both the infestation and the causative conditions to a level at which they no longer have an adverse effect on the community.

Interventions: Actions taken to prevent, reduce, or eliminate rodent infestations and their destructive effects. Survey data determine when, where, what, and whether interventions are necessary to prevent or eliminate a particular pest problem. Interventions are classified as educational, legal or regulatory, habitat modification, horticultural, biologic, mechanical, and chemical. These intervention categories typically form an IPM strategy. Most commensal rodent IPM programs emphasize educational and legal or regulatory interventions, and habitat modification.

The key to a successful IPM program is the elimination of the causes of infestation (i.e., food, water, and harborage). The judicious and careful use of pesticides (including toxicants) to manage pests is also important for success. A vital IPM "rule" for selecting rodenticides or other pesticides is that the product chosen should be the least toxic product that will be effective on a target pest. The product also must have a highly efficacious and readily available antidote that can be administered in a timely manner for both humans and pets if a rodenticide is inadvertently ingested. Widespread and indiscriminate use of pesticides, a problem Rachel Carson warned about in her 1967 book *Silent Spring*, has serious consequences for people, animals, and the environment.

Evaluation: The evaluation process (composed of periodic surveys) determines whether IPM interventions have been effective or whether they need to be repeated or modified. The initial survey of residential and commercial blocks and the periodic resurveys (monitoring) of a target community provides the basis for the evaluation of a program's progress.

Characteristics of Urban Rodent Surveys

A health-related government agency or department typically manages a community-based vector control program. For the purpose of this manual, such agencies or organizations will be referred to as the "IPM authority." The responsible adult, whether a homeowner or a renter, who grants permission to inspect a premises or dwelling will be called the "householder."

The initial urban rodent survey is the data gathering phase of IPM program planning. Conducting the survey provides the IPM authority with an opportunity to inform residents about the program and to encourage their support when survey teams inspect their premises. An analysis of survey results will show the extent and severity of rodent infestations and their causative conditions and will delineate IPM program needs as well as the progress made in comparison with previous surveys.

To determine the magnitude of the rodent problem, determine priorities, and evaluate progress, the IPM program must maintain a premises and block records management system. The system should provide for sequentially reporting survey findings using standardized reporting forms.

The urban rodent survey involves an exterior inspection of premises to record significant data such as active rodent signs, rodent entries to buildings, and environmental deficiencies that provide food, water, and harborage. Although the Norway rat and the roof rat generally live outdoors, they do enter buildings that are not rodent proofed. The house mouse can survive outdoors, but it prefers indoor areas in an urban habitat. Whenever rodents find suitable food, water, and harborage, they become established and reproduce rapidly. Interior inspections of dwellings and buildings may be required if signs of infestation are obvious. Gaining access to interiors of premises is, however, generally more difficult, and the problems associated with the management and control of interior infestations are greater. Nevertheless, interior inspection is considered an essential component of an IPM program if clear evidence exists of significant interior infestation.

Two forms are required for an exterior urban rodent survey: a field inspection form and a summary form for office tabulations (Appendix A, Figures 1–4; Figures 1 and 3 are blank forms and Figures 2 and 4 are completed examples). These forms can be modified to serve the special needs of local programs. Although the use of check marks on a form may suffice to indicate the presence of deficiencies on premises, some programs use a coding system (e.g., letters, numbers, colors) to record more detailed information. Examples of such codes are furnished throughout this manual as an alternative to the checkmark system.

The survey forms provide the necessary data to plan and conduct a rodent IPM program. These data identify the need for rodent proofing, code enforcement, refuse management, cleanup of vacant lots, removal of abandoned automobiles and appliances, and other necessary interventions. The IPM approach emphasizes site-specific combinations of interventions to control or eliminate rodent populations.

In a more detailed version of the survey, a third form can be added for interior inspections. This form can be modified from the exterior inspection form to provide detailed data for each area or room within residential or commercial premises. This detailed information is useful in two ways: in determining where rodents may frequent and nest in particular areas of a premises or dwelling and in assessing rodent-related risks such as the potential for bites or food contamination.

Basic Units in the Operational Program

For planning, operating, and reporting purposes, all rodent IPM programs use basic geographic units such as the following:

1. **Premises** (to record existing conditions). A premises is a plot of land with or without a building. It is the basic unit of a program in which survey items can be observed and recorded (e.g., environmental deficiencies, active rodent signs). Maintenance of a premises is usually the responsibility of a householder (unless multiple dwelling units are on a premises), superintendent, or manager who must maintain the environmental quality of the premises. For survey purposes, all premises are classified as residential, commercial, commercial and residential, or vacant lot. Schools, parks, churches, and parking areas are defined as commercial.

   A premises may consist of an individual residence and its surroundings—whether attached (e.g., row house) or detached (e.g., a stand-alone home). A duplex house or a large apartment building and its surroundings are considered a single premises because they are usually under one ownership and are situated on one plot of land. The same criteria apply to a commercial premises with a major building and other structures. For larger aggregations of buildings, such as several apartment buildings under one or several ownerships, each numbered building and its surroundings are considered to be a separate premises. Reviewing municipal tax parcel maps may be helpful to clarify the physical (e.g., property lines) and administrative (e.g., ownership) data related to a particular property. Where available, use of a geographic information system (GIS) to map properties can be helpful.

2. **Block** (to classify conditions). The block is a convenient unit for reporting infestations and causative conditions, recording interventions, and determining progress. In a target community, premises information should be aggregated for each block and filed according to assigned block numbers. A block is reported as infested as long as any active rodent signs exist on a single premises.

   A block is ordinarily bounded by four streets, but some blocks are bounded by three or fewer, or may be irregular in form. In some cases, imaginary boundaries conforming to prevailing block sizes may be set to define a block.

3. **Census Tract** (multiple contiguous blocks). The census tract is an excellent unit for large-scale planning and reporting purposes. Some IPM authorities use zones, wards, or elementary school or health districts for reporting purposes.

4. **Target Area** (entire operational area of an IPM program). Large cities may have several target areas.

Sample Versus Comprehensive Surveys

The block survey is considered comprehensive if all premises in all blocks in a defined target area are surveyed. In a sample survey, all premises on a block are inspected in a small but statistically valid number of blocks in a defined target area. Comprehensive surveys provide complete information on rodent infestation and sanitary conditions in a defined target area. Sample surveys are appropriate for defining an infestation problem and its causative conditions for a target area, but they are not appropriate for intervention purposes.

The sample survey is quicker to do than a comprehensive survey because all premises are inspected only within a randomly selected sample of the blocks in the proposed or actual target area. This type of survey is typically used to determine the need for a rodent IPM program; to define program needs and requirements for personnel, material, and equipment; and to later evaluate program progress.

Sample surveys are not intended for citywide application, although exceptions exist. Sample surveys are valuable for determining potential target areas. After a sample survey is completed, a comprehensive survey needs to be conducted. Potential target areas often are identified by number and location of rodent complaints, reported rodent bites, deteriorating housing conditions, and other related indicators including causative conditions of infestation.

A comprehensive survey requires significantly more personnel than a sample survey, but it has considerably greater impact on the community because all premises in the target area are inspected. Comprehensive surveys should be conducted concurrently with public education, community outreach, code enforcement, neighborhood cleanup campaigns, and other IPM activities. Two comprehensive surveys are recommended per target area per year. More frequent surveys are desirable, but resource considerations can be a limiting factor.

Personnel Requirements

Ideally, urban rodent surveys should be conducted by two-person teams, with the most qualified person recording the data and making decisions about questionable findings. Safety is also a factor in a team approach.

Survey teams, where possible, should be composed of experienced rodent control specialists, environmental health specialists, or other trained personnel. Knowledge of the area to be surveyed, when practical, can also be helpful, especially if a member of the survey team lives in the area to be surveyed. The survey teams should be guided by the exterior inspection form, which is to be completed during the inspection.

At least 3 to 5 days of classroom and field training are recommended for inspectors to ensure that their observational and recordkeeping skills are satisfactory. To conduct interior inspections, additional classroom and field training is necessary.

IPM surveys are a detail-dependent process. The number of premises inspected per team per day will vary with experience, complexity of the built environment, and other variables. For example, large lots, multiple dwellings on a premises, difficult-to-access alleys, and complex building designs need to be considered in determining the time required to conduct a survey.

In most communities, permission for entry onto premises must be obtained before conducting an inspection. People may resent the intrusion onto their properties unless they understand and accept the purpose of the inspections. Community support should be sought to enhance program success. This support can be gained by meeting with community representatives, church groups, and others in advance of the survey.

Survey Procedures

Conducting an urban rodent survey involves four phases: preparation, public information and education, inspection, and analysis.

1. **Preparation**. *Planning the operation and recruiting and training staff.* Provision should be made to secure official photo identification cards and distinctive uniforms to identify field staff. Vehicles that are clearly marked with the IPM or department logo will enhance the community's perception of the program. Vehicles are used to transport inspection staff, materials, and supplies for intervention purposes.

2. **Public Information and Education**. *Using communication materials to promote the IPM program.* Agencies or department officials should use news media, Web sites, exhibits, and brochures and posters as well as visit the target area to inform residents in advance of the survey and explain its importance. There should be outreach to community organizations, parent-teacher associations, churches, building manager associations, trade unions, and other groups to gain support for the program. Contact should also be established with local official agencies (e.g., housing, sanitation, sewer, utilities) and others who may have interest in or responsibilities associated with the program.

These contacts can be invaluable in the planning and implementation process. In addition, accommodation for residents who work during the day needs to be built into the program's work schedule. This accommodation may sometimes require that those working in public education and outreach activities will have to work in the early evenings or on weekends.

3. **Inspection**. *Inspecting premises for active rodent signs (e.g., droppings, rub marks, open burrows) and causative conditions (e.g., improper refuse storage, pet food) in target areas and recording data on the exterior inspection form (Appendix A, Figure 1).* Evaluation is an essential component of the survey process. Taking photographs can be helpful in understanding particular infestation problems and can be used for training purposes is part of the evaluation process. Although inspections are generally conducted during daylight hours, we recommend that senior staff occasionally visit the target area at night to view conditions during the rodents' active period. These night inspections will add clarity to the relation between the rodents and their built environment. They will also provide a better understanding of the impact of poor refuse management. Infrared video cameras can be used to document rodent activity at night.

4. **Analysis**. *Tabulating findings, analyzing data, and comparing achievements.* Analysis of data provides the basis for developing work plans and for preparing reports with recommendations for eliminating infestations. Such reports often are supplemented by tables, graphs, maps, and photographs.

Sample Survey Methodology

Initiating a sample survey requires maps, survey forms, and complete lists of blocks or premises of the target area. Each premises must be clearly defined and given a number so that it can be unambiguously identified on the map. Because of expected variations in block configurations, decide what constitutes a block for survey purposes. All field personnel must be aware of that definition.

The procedure for selecting the sample number of blocks for a random block survey follows:

1. Determine as closely as possible the number of blocks and premises within the target area or areas to be surveyed.

2. Determine the number of premises that will have to be inspected to ensure statistical validity (Table 1). Note: Sample sizes must adhere to the minimum standards; the reliability of the survey results depends on adherence to the standards.

3. Divide the number of blocks in a target area into the estimated number of premises. The equation below represents the average number of premises per block in the target area.

$$\text{Example:} \quad \frac{20{,}000 \text{ premises}}{1{,}000 \text{ blocks}} = 20 \text{ premises per block}$$

4. Determine the number of blocks so that a sufficient number of premises (as obtained from Table 1) will be surveyed.

Example: If at least 500 premises need to be inspected, and the target area contains an average of 25 premises per block, then all premises on 20 blocks will need to be surveyed.

$$\frac{500 \text{ premises needed}}{25 \text{ (average premises per block)}} = 20 \text{ blocks}$$

5. Select the 20 blocks by using a table of random numbers (Appendix B, Table B-1), with each number representing a specific numbered block.

Note: When using this method, every premises on a selected block should be inspected, even if repeat visits are required.

Another survey method is to randomly select a sample of premises in the target area for inspection. For this method, a complete list of premises is needed, but such a list can be difficult to obtain. This particular method requires assigning every premises a number and identifying each premises on a map.

Survey Crews and Equipment

Two-person teams are more efficient to conduct block surveys. Each team should carry the following items:

- a supply of field forms (exterior, interior, or both, depending on the needs of the program),

- mechanical lead pencils and lead refills (0.5-millimeter leads, HB type),

- clipboards,

- flashlights (rechargeable type is recommended),

- gloves,

- forceps,

- hand lenses (5–10X),

- small plastic vials and zip-close plastic bags for field samples (e.g., dead rodent specimens, fecal droppings),

- black light to detect rodent urine stains,

- dog repellent,

- digital still cameras, and

- mobile phones or pagers (for communication between supervisors and inspection teams and for emergency situations).

Table 1. Minimum Number of Premises Inspected to Ensure Statistical Validity*	
Number of Premises in Target Area	Minimum Number of Premises to Inspect
10,000 or more	500
3,000–9,999	450
Up to 2,999	435
*Center for Disease Control. Urban rat surveys. Atlanta: US Department of Health and Human Services; 1974.	

Note that a personal digital assistant (PDA) can be used instead of the field forms, lead pencils, and clipboards. Also note that infrared video cameras can be a valuable tool for filming rodents at night.

For indoor inspections, add the following items:

- small and large flashlights (headlamps, if practical),

- extendable inspection mirrors,

- dust masks or respirators,

- hard hats,

- portable vacuum cleaners with high-efficiency particulate air (HEPA) filters, and

- small ladders (4 feet [1.2 meters]).

If a recording code (instead of a check mark) is to be used on the forms for more precise information about specific data categories, a copy of the codes should be taped to the clipboard for easy reference. The inspection forms can be relatively simple or can be greatly detailed depending on the needs of the survey. Inspection forms can be completed using PDAs and other portable computer equipment.

Each team should have a supply of outreach literature on the program to distribute to landlords and householders during the surveys.

Premises Inspection—Exterior

Supervisors should hand out the block assignments before the teams leave the office. For multiple teams, the supervisor should remain in the immediate area to monitor the work of the teams and to provide support as needed.

A standardized survey process is more effective; for example, begin the survey of each block at the northeast corner and move clockwise. From this corner, the inspectors proceed around the block, inspecting each premises in the order established for the survey. The two-member teams may work together on an inspection, or, if both are experienced, they may inspect alternate primeses and be available to assist each other as needed. Placing a chalk mark on the curb after a primeses has been inspected can be useful if a supervisor needs to locate the team; however, inspectors may use portable phones to maintain contact.

Each premises should be approached from its main entrance area and should not be entered by crossing yards. The inspector should request permission from a responsible adult to conduct an inspection. A brochure that explains the program can supplement the explanation of the program and the purpose of the inspection. Usually, only a few minutes are required to communicate effectively with householders. Occupants of the premises should be encouraged to join in the survey of the premises. This participation allows inspectors an opportunity to praise occupants for the well-maintained aspects of the primeses, such as a clean yard, and to tactfully call attention to active rodent signs or sanitation deficiencies.

Inspectors should wear clear identification that identifies them as a representative of the rodent IPM program. Wearing distinctive official uniforms also can be helpful in establishing identity with the program.

Before proceeding with the exterior inspection of a premises, write the number of dwelling units on the exterior inspection form (Appendix A, Figure 1, column 7. See the Instructions for Completing the Block Record (Exterior Inspection) Form section on pages FILL). The team should then proceed in a clockwise direction around the premises, inspecting the buildings, yard, and passageway(s) or other spaces, and recording all deficiencies on the survey form. The inspection pattern is as follows:

- front (the facade or surface of the building that contains the main entrance and its associated yard or other spaces),

- left side (left wall surface of building and its associated yard or other spaces),

- back or rear (the rear wall surface of the building and its associated yard or other spaces), and

- right side (the right wall surface of the building and its associated yard or other spaces).

Symbols can be used instead of check marks to record information. These symbols can also be used as a reference in the Remarks section or in the premises

Address column of the form; for example, F: front (with main entrance to building), L: left side, B: back or rear, and R: right side.

Rodent signs should be observed at close range to determine infestation. Inspectors should look for active rodent runs or burrows in the yard, entry routes into buildings, burrows under walls or in ditch banks, rodent damage, fresh fecal droppings along foundations, and other evidence of infestation.

Before leaving a premises, inspectors should check the inspection form to make certain that all items have been completed. Having a supervisor or another field inspector recheck the survey findings on a subsequent day to verify results can be helpful (e.g., taking a 10% sample of the surveyed premises to ensure the recorded information is accurate and complete).

In some instances, householders may refuse permission for IPM staff to inspect their premises or dwelling. These refusals should be noted on the report form and referred to the supervisor. In other instances, no responsible adult may be at home to grant permission for inspection. In such cases, the policy of the IPM authority determines whether to conduct the exterior inspection.

Premises Inspection—Interior

The term "interior inspection" generally applies to the main buildings on a premises and not to sheds or outbuildings (this delineation can be modified to meet the needs of the local IPM authority). Two-person teams are recommended for interior inspections. The work is detail-oriented, tedious, and often difficult to accomplish because of clutter, furniture, and crowded conditions.

Inspectors should check all rooms in the building for rodent signs and sanitation deficiencies. Kitchens, closets, bathrooms, attics, and basements are especially attractive to commensal rodents. All floor levels of the building should be inspected regardless of the suspected species. Norway rats are usually found in basements and on lower floors; upper floors and attic areas are especially attractive to roof rats; and house mice can be found nearly anywhere, including in cabinet drawers and above drop ceilings. Householders often can be helpful in providing specific information on a rodent infestation.

In some communities, the interior rodent population may be more difficult to manage or control than the exterior population. The exterior inspection form (Appendix A, Figure 1) can be modified for interior inspections. When doing so, information such as level/floor, room type, and number of occupants as well as information on active rodent signs (droppings, holes, gnawed materials, and rub marks) should be included on the modified form. Information about rodent bites should also be collected.

Infestation rates (i.e., percent of apartments in a building with active rodent signs) are useful in comparing conditions or measuring IPM progress over time.

Inspection teams should follow standardized procedures for interior inspections. For example, in a multifamily apartment building, start in the basement, then work upward, inspecting apartments in numerical order, then inspect the attic or crawlspace, and finally the roof (if accessible). Enter each apartment through the front (main) door and inspect the wall that contains the main door as well as everything on or touching that wall for signs of rodents and potential rodent entries. Move clockwise to the next wall and continue until all walls are inspected. Next, inspect the floor area, including anything on or touching the floor. Last, inspect the ceiling area, including anything on or touching the ceiling. Each room should be inspected in the same manner. Closets should be inspected in association with particular walls of a room.

This standardized inspection method provides very specific data on rodent locations for intervention purposes. The data also simplify the tracking of specific changes over time and provide information for other inspectors.

Instructions for Completing the Block Record (Exterior Inspection) Form

The Block Record—Exterior Rodent Inspection and Sanitation Form (Appendix A, Figure 1) is used to record information on rodent infestation and environmental deficiencies for each premises on a block. The form has space for recording information for 10 premises; additional forms can be used as necessary. Enter the page number in the space provided at the top right corner of the form (i.e., "1 of 2," "2 of 2"). If only one form is required for a block, use the same notation (i.e., "1 of 1") to clarify that only one page is required. In addition, enter the names of the inspectors at the top of the form in the space provided.

Other items at the top of the form should be completed by the supervisor or team leader before the teams enter entering the field. The location of a block should be indicated by writing the names of the streets that form the block in the block diagram space in the upper left portion of the form.

A copy of the assignment chart should be kept in the inspector's or supervisor's office.

Completed inspection forms (Appendix A, Figure 2) should be checked and initialed by the inspectors. All columns of block data should be totaled and recorded on the appropriate line of the summary form (Appendix A, Figure 4 is a completed example). The summary form should be used to prepare progress reports, identify problems, and target resources.

Premises Address

- As inspectors proceed clockwise around a block, they should write each street address in the left column. If an indoor inspection has been conducted at a particular address, the line number (1 to 10) in the "No." column should be circled.

Premises Type

A premises must be classified in one of four categories (columns 1–4): residential, commercial and residential, commercial, or vacant lot. Only one of the first four columns should be checked.

Column 1: Residential

Put a check in this column if the unit is a home or dwelling (defined as an enclosed space used for living purposes). A dwelling can be a single-family or multifamily unit. Enter the number of dwelling units in column 7 (No. of Dwelling Units).

Column 2: Commercial and Residential

Put a check in this column if a premises is used for both commercial (see column 3 description) and residential purposes.

Column 3: Commercial

Put a check in this column if the premises is used only for commercial purposes (including parking lots) or for other nonresidential purposes such as offices, churches, clubhouses, or schools. The type of premises (e.g., school) may also be written in the address column. Some IPM programs may decide to use a code for recording public properties, clubs, churches, or other types of nonresidential properties.

Column 4: Vacant Lot

Put a check in this column for a lot with no structure on it. Note that a parking lot should be designated as "commercial."

Premises Details

Use these four columns of the inspection form to record information that may be helpful in estimating population density and in determining resource needs for intervention purposes.

Column 5: Food-Commercial

Put a check in this column if a regular, primary function of the premises is to prepare, sell, serve or dispense, or store food materials, including animal foods. Thus, restaurants, delicatessens, soup kitchens, bakeries, grocery stores, nursing homes and hospitals (where daily meals are served), pet stores, and grain warehouses should be included here. Both this column and column 2 or 3 should be checked.

Column 6: Vacant

Put a check in this column if the main building on the premises is not in use, whether temporarily vacant, permanently abandoned, or boarded up and scheduled for demolition. Abandoned buildings generally are not considered habitable because of deterioration (e.g., broken windows, missing doors, vandalism, fire damage). If more precise information is desired, three symbols can be used in this column instead of a check mark: V: vacant and habitable, AO: abandoned and open, and AS: abandoned and sealed.

Column 7: No. of Dwelling Units

Enter the number of dwelling units here. Determining the number of dwelling units on a premises should be based on the following definition:

A dwelling unit is a room or group of rooms located within a building or structure that forms a single habitable unit to be used for living, sleeping, cooking, and eating.

Multiple dwelling units (e.g., apartments) can exist on a premises. The number of mailboxes, meters, or doorbells is an indicator of the number of dwelling units on a premises. Only the number of habitable dwelling units on a premises should be marked; non-inhabitable dwelling units should not be marked.

Column 8: Sewers on Premises

Put a check in this column to record the presence of a sewer pipes or storm water drains on the premises. Sewers can provide harborage, and rats often travel between a premises sewer and the exterior portions of the premises. Evidence of harborage includes active burrows near manholes, catch basins, or broken sewer pipes, and fresh rub marks on broken downspouts that empty into sewers. If other sewer deficiencies are found, do not check them; use an asterisk and include a footnote under the Remarks section of the form.

Food

These columns (numbers 9–12) provide information on food sources that must be eliminated.

Proper storage of refuse (also called municipal solid waste or MSW) requires the use of rodent-proof containers of adequate construction, size, and number. Refuse is defined as a mixture of garbage and rubbish. Garbage consists largely of human food waste (organic, putrescible), but it includes offal, carrion, and animal feces (e.g., dog or horse). Rubbish is considered nonfood solid wastes (combustible and noncombustible, nonputrescible) such as metal, glass, furniture, carpeting, paper, and cardboard. Rubbish also includes wood chips and yard wastes.

In conducting rodent surveys, the following criteria for refuse storage are recommended.

Approved Refuse Storage

- Refuse containers should be water tight with tight fitting lids that may be hinged; rust resistant; structurally strong; and easily filled, emptied, and cleaned. Standard refuse containers are 20–32 gallons (91–150 liters). Hinged containers with wheels can hold up to 95 gallons (430 liters). Bulk containers such as dumpsters have side handles or bail for manual handling or special attachment hooks and devices for automatic or semiautomatic handling.

- Bulk storage containers are generally acceptable and are often used in multihousing buildings, commercial establishments, and construction sites. Such containers often have a drain hole to facilitate cleaning. These drain holes are often 2–3 inches (5–8 centimeters) in diameter and are fitted with a removable hardware cloth screen or screw-on plug to prevent entry by rodents.

- Galvanized metal or heavy, high-grade plastic containers meet the guidelines under a in the Column 10 section.

- Cardboard boxes used for yard trash (essentially nonfood items) are acceptable.

- Plastic or moisture resistant paper bags used for refuse, properly tied and intact, placed at the curb or alley only on collection day and only during daylight hours are acceptable.

Plastic Bags

Plastic refuse bags are widely used as liners in standard 20–32 gallon (91–150 liters) and larger refuse containers. These bags are required by many building managers for refuse placed in bulk containers and are used by many residents for yard trash.

To judge whether plastic bags are managed properly:

- Know the scheduled refuse collection days in the block being surveyed.

- Observe whether the storage site contains both acceptable bags and refuse containers or whether plastic bags appear to be the sole containers for storing refuse.

Plastic bags are not considered appropriate for overnight storage outdoors because nocturnally active rodents and other animals (e.g., cats, dogs) can easily gain access to their contents. Plastic bags should be considered acceptable only when placed outside during daylight hours for collection the same day.

Approved Recyclable Storage

- Outdoor containers for recyclable items (paper, cardboard, plastic, glass, or metal cans) should be water-tight, strong enough to support the weight of items contained, and easy for sanitation crews to handle.

- Containers similar to those for refuse storage are generally acceptable for household recyclables, as are large plastic bags properly tied and intact and placed at the curb or alley only during daylight hours on collection day.

- In all cases, items stored should be free of food particles or other food residue.

To judge whether recyclables are managed properly:

- Know the scheduled recyclable collection days for the block being surveyed.

- Observe whether the recyclable items have been cleaned or rinsed or are otherwise free of food residue and that the plastic bags or other containers holding the recyclables are intact.

Column 9: Unapproved Refuse Storage

Put a check in this column if garbage, rubbish, other refuse, or recyclable items are not stored in approved containers with tight fitting lids (or are not in tightly tied bags—where acceptable—during daytime only). Approved containers should be of the design described in the Approved Refuse Storage section. When properly placed in plastic or paper bags, securely tied, and regularly collected, yard trash and other inedible materials are approved. Yard trash is acceptable when placed in cardboard boxes or paper bags and regularly collected.

Put a check in this column if any of the following conditions are observed:

- Container that is not rodent and fly tight.

- Screw-on plug or rodent-excluding screen of

an otherwise approved bulk container is not in place or is missing.

- 55 gallon (250-liter) drum. Such containers are often observed without a tight-fitting cover. When filled, they are too heavy and bulky to handle.

- Nonstandard metal or cardboard containers that are not being used for regularly collected yard trash.

- Bin or stationary receptacle for refuse storage.

- Receptacle too small or too few receptacles for the amount of refuse.

- Overflowing receptacle or one with the cover off.

- Container(s) on a platform on the ground or with a shallow space (<18 inches [46 centimeters] high) that offers harborage for rodents and possibly hides scraps of food spilled from the container.

- Burned refuse.

- Scattered refuse (including garbage, rubbish, or recyclables).

More-precise information can be obtained by using symbols instead of check marks to record specific deficiencies.

Column 10: Exposed Garbage

Put a check in this column if observed refuse storage practices make garbage available to rodents. In many cases, a premises may be noted for Unapproved Refuse Storage, but no garbage available to rodents is observed. Exposed garbage should be noted on the basis of the following:

a. Garbage container is not rodent tight (the space between the container and lid is greater than ¼ inch [0.64 centimeters], and the container is used for garbage storage).

b. Garbage in an open container is available to rodents.

c. Garbage is scattered on the ground. Plastic bags containing garbage are ripped, present after dark, not properly tied, or have obviously not been collected for longer than 1 day. Clean beer cans, soft-drink bottles, and old food cans and jars are not considered a rodent food source. **Note: Vegetable and fruit plants are recorded under Other Food and Plants, not as Exposed Garbage. Any premises marked for Exposed Garbage should also be marked for Unapproved Refuse Storage.**

Column 11: Animal Food

Put a check here if uneaten animal food (e.g., food for pets such as dogs or cats, birds, or livestock) is exposed outdoors or if it is exposed in an outbuilding accessible to rodents. Exposed pet food, other than for immediate feeding, should be recorded. In the case of birdfeeders, check only if uneaten birdseed is observed on the ground and is readily available to rodents. However, some commensal rodents are excellent climbers, so caution should be exercised in assessing birdfeeders. Animal food should not be recorded as exposed garbage.

Column 12: Other Food and Plants

Put a check in this column if vegetables, fruit and nut trees, or ornamental shrubs and vines with fruits and berries are accessible to rodents. Put a check in this column if exposed food items in the dwelling's interior are observed but are not easily classified in the other four columns. Items for this column include soiled dishes exposed overnight, food waste on the stove or in the oven, and solid or liquid foods on the floor.

Water

Although commensal rodent dependency on water varies with diet and species, water sources should be eliminated. High-protein diets increase a rodent's need for water, but house mice are capable of living with little water. All three species (Norway rat, roof rat, and house mouse), however, are attracted to water when it is available. Natural bodies of water, such as streams, lakes, and ponds, are excluded from the survey. The three survey categories in the Water section (columns 13–15) are observable water resources that need to be managed as part of IPM habitat modification interventions. Only one of the three columns should be checked for water available to rodents.

Water and moisture reduction can also enhance IPM practices to control mosquitoes, cockroaches, and mold (especially indoors).

Column 13: Standing Water

Put a check in this column if water accumulations that are accessible to rodents are found in containers such as buckets, pans, discarded tires, water bowls for pets, window pits of basements, and clogged rain gutters. For indoor inspections, check for water and other consumable liquids that are available overnight in open containers on tables or desks or in sinks, cooking pans, and buckets.

Column 14: Condensate

Put a check in this column if condensate is available to rodents in, for example, collection pans under refrigeration or air conditioning units; from dripping or running water from a pipe onto the ground or pavement (or onto a basement floor indoors); or directly from the surface of, or dripping from, cold water pipes indoors.

Column 15: Leaks

Put a check in this column if water is regularly leaking from, for example, a roof, pipe, or outdoor faucet onto the ground, pavement, or floor (indoors). For observed leaks, do not check the Standing Water category even if water has accumulated.

Harborage

The seven survey items in this section (columns 16–22) pertain to the providing of harborage for rodents. Put a check in any column only if the inspector judges that a significant rodent harborage condition is evident. For some surveys, quantifying the harborage present is helpful (e.g., using figures to indicate the number of abandoned vehicles and appliances or to estimate the number of cubic yards or cubic meters of large piles of rubbish, lumber, or clutter that is on the ground or on the floor indoors). These figures can be useful in estimating the resources needed for cleanup and for measuring progress in reducing the amount of harborage present.

Column 16: Abandoned Vehicles

Put a check in this column if abandoned vehicles are in the yard, street, or alley. A vehicle is considered abandoned if the license tag is not current, if major parts are missing, or if high grass and weeds are growing around it. Abandoned vehicles observed in rodent-accessible garages should also be recorded. The summary line at the bottom of the form should note the number of premises with abandoned vehicles. The total number of vehicles may be entered directly below the column total if vehicles are counted for each premises.

Column 17: Abandoned Appliances

Put a check in this column if appliances (such as refrigerators, stoves, or washing machines) are stored in the yard, in a dilapidated outbuilding, or at the edge of an adjoining street or alley. Put only one check mark regardless of the number of items observed; however, the number of appliances may be entered in the column instead of a check mark. The survey summary line should show the number of premises with abandoned appliances, not the number of appliances. The total number of appliances may be entered directly below the column total if appliances are counted for each premises.

Column 18: Lumber or Clutter on the Ground

Put a check in this column if a significant amount (covering at least 1 square yard or 1 square meter) of lumber, firewood, or clutter is on the ground. These materials provide harborage for rodents. Clutter, either outdoors or indoors, is defined as disorganized storage of usable materials (not rubbish) that is not being used and which impedes inspections for active rodent infestation. A few scattered pieces of lumber or other materials should not be recorded, nor should lumber left on the ground as a result of recent building construction or demolition and is subject to early removal. If the amount is to be quantified, estimate the number of cubic yards (or cubic meters) to the nearest whole number. The number recorded in the Total row at the bottom of the column, however, is always the total number of premises with a deficiency. The total number of cubic yards (or cubic meters) of lumber or clutter may be entered directly below the column total for premises.

Column 19: Other Large Rubbish

In both exterior and interior inspections, put a check in this column if there are discarded items of rubbish that are too large or otherwise not suitable for storage in approved refuse containers. These items include tires, automobile engines, large cans and drums, tree limbs, rubble, doors, mattresses, furniture, and other large items not listed in other columns. If the amount is to be quantified, estimate the number of cubic yards (or cubic meters) to the nearest whole number and enter the number directly below the column total.

Column 20: Outbuildings or Privies

Put a check in this column only if the buildings on the premises are dilapidated or otherwise provide significant rodent harborage. A tight, well maintained building or an open, clean shed should not be recorded. Appliances, lumber, clutter, or large rubbish in an open shed should be reported in their respective columns if they furnish harborage. Always check this column when privies or outhouses are found.

Column 21: Board Fences and Walls

Put a check in this column if dilapidated board fences, walls, or concrete slabs (e.g., patio slabs, broken sidewalks) are found because they can provide harborage for rodents.

Column 22: Plant-Related

Put a check in this column if weeds or grass are more than 12 inches (0.3 meters) high and are sufficiently thick to hide refuse and provide harborage for rodents. Bushes and overgrown shrubbery that provide rodent harborage are also deficiencies that should be recorded. Note that roof rats are climbers and prefer to nest in trees, bushes, and attics of dwellings and outbuildings. Put a check mark in this column if dense growth such as ivy, honeysuckle, pyracantha, ground cover, dense shrubbery or vines, or palm trees provide harborage for rodents. Large planters indoors or outdoors may provide harborage for rodents, either in the soil or among dense vegetation. If more precise information is desired, symbols identifying types of dense growth may be used to record such deficiencies.

Entry and Access

The two columns in this section (columns 23–24) are for recording the need for rodent-stoppage work to prevent rodents from entering structures.

A Norway rat can gain access to a structure through a hole the diameter of a U.S. quarter (0.96 inches or 24.3 millimeters in diameter) and a mouse can gain access through a hole the diameter of a U.S. dime (0.71 inches or 17.9 millimeters in diameter). Structural openings should be less than ¾-inch (<19 millimeters) in diameter to exclude adult Norway rats, less than ½-inch (<13 millimeters) in diameter to exclude adult roof rats, and less than ¼-in (<6 millimeters) in diameter to exclude adult mice. If openings are sealed (totally closed), cockroaches and other insects will also be excluded.

From a running start, a house mouse can jump up to 2 feet (0.6 meters) high, a Norway rat up to 3 feet (0.9 meters) high, and a roof rat up to 4 feet (1.2 meters) high. Therefore, openings up to 5 feet (1.5 meters) from the ground must be sealed or covered with mesh.

Column 23: Structural Deficiencies

Put a check in this column if an actual or potential rodent entry to a building because of deterioration or structural defects is observed. Common defects include holes in crumbling masonry foundations, deteriorated fascia boards at the edge of roofs, and poorly fitted doors with gaps of sufficient size to permit rodent entry.

Column 24: Pipe and Wiring Gaps

Check this column to indicate that a gap or hole associated with a wire, pipe, or other conduit penetrates the building exterior (including basement floor or roof) and is sufficiently large to permit rodent entry. For indoor inspections, check this column if openings in interior walls, floors, or ceilings are found.

Active Signs

Put a check in column 25 if active or fresh rodent signs are observed during exterior or interior inspections. A premises is considered infested with rodents only if active signs are found (e.g., sightings, droppings, runways, rub marks, burrows or openings, gnaw marks,

tracks). The infestation rate is calculated on the basis of the number of premises on a block with active rodent signs divided by the total number of premises on a block times 100.

If additional details are desired, symbols could be placed in or next to the column to distinguish signs attributable to Norway rats, roof rats, or house mice. Active rodent signs usually will be one or more of the signs listed below. More precise information can be recorded by using the following symbols instead of check marks:

B. Burrows: active burrow entrances do not have cobwebs or other blockages.

D. Fecal droppings or urine: fresh feces are dark and soft; old feces are hard or gray and brittle; urine may be wet, glossy, or sticky or may be a dried stain. A black light can help show rodent urine stains.

H. Gnawed holes, gnaw marks, or tooth marks: a freshly gnawed surface is usually light in color.

M. Rub marks: if fresh, they are black, soft, and greasy.

R. Runs: well traveled paths (Note: runs usually lead to food sources, water, and harborage).

T. Tracks: fresh foot tracks or tail-drag marks.

Z. Rodent hairs: often found on rub marks or at entry holes to buildings.

Remarks

This section at the bottom of the form is for additional information.

Interior Inspection Using a Modified Block Record (Exterior Inspection) Form

Much of the methodology for completing an interior inspection is the same or similar to that for an exterior inspection. A modified interior inspection form focuses exclusively on deficiencies found indoors. An interior form should include space for the premises address and the number of dwelling units at that address. The form's design should depend on the needs of the local

IPM program, but suggested categories are listed in this section. Many of these categories are explained in the Instructions for Completing the Block Record (Exterior Inspection) Form; categories not explained in that section are explained below.

Premises Type

- residential,

- commercial and residential, and

- commercial.

Premises Details

- level or floor (where unit is located),

- room type (e.g., bedroom, bathroom, hallway, kitchen),

- number of occupants in unit, and

- sewer pipes or storm water drains on premises.

Food

- unapproved refuse storage,

- exposed garbage,

- animal food,

- unapproved food storage (food material stored in open or unprotected boxes, bags, bins, or other containers or stored under storage conditions that are not rodent proof [e.g., cereal cartons]), and

- other food and plants.

Water

- standing water,

- condensate, and

- plumbing leaks.

Harborage

- clutter or storage on the floor,

- other large rubbish,

- plant-related, and

- other harborage (small accumulations of material that may be viewed as providing harborage [e.g., piles of clothes on the floor]).

Entry and Access

- structural deficiencies and

- pipe and wiring gaps

Active Signs

- fecal droppings, urine;

- holes, gnawings, burrows;

- tracks, runs, rub marks; and

- rodent bites reported (This item is to capture information on whether the occupant has reported being bitten by a rodent within the 6-month period before the inspection. Information should be collected about the demographics of the victim, the biting incident, and the action taken by the health authority. Information about the rodent infestation, bites, circumstances, unsanitary conditions, food and water access, and harborage will be valuable in the effort to eliminate the infestation.

Note: Having the inspection team carry a small portable HEPA-filtering vacuum cleaner to remove rodent signs (e.g., droppings and nesting material) may be beneficial. The vacuum cleaner can also be used to remove potentially allergenic material from the dwelling.

Remarks

The modified interior inspection form should also include a Remarks section to record additional information (e.g., heavy rat infestation in an apartment with very young children) that requires immediate attention or referral to another department.

GIS and Mapping

GIS is a highly valued tool, as are maps of the target area or community. Maps help define the infestation problem and its causes as well as measure progress toward eliminating the problem. Maps of the target area are often used by programs to make block inspection assignments, show changing patterns in infestations and their causative conditions, and measure progress in addressing the rodent problem. Table 2 shows examples of the types of major deficiencies and associated map colors on a GIS map.

Maps may be prepared for other causative conditions, including water sources and entry and access routes. These maps can be used as a tool to determine priorities for corrective actions.

The goal of an IPM program should be to reduce rodent populations and their causative conditions to a level that they no longer have an adverse effect on the community. The following set of criteria should be achieved for a block or for the defined target area:

**2% or less of the premises
with active exterior rodent signs and either
15% or less of the premises
with exposed garbage,
or
30% or less of the premises with
unapproved refuse storage.**

These criteria are based on those used by the federal urban rat control program directed by CDC from 1972 to 1981 throughout the United States. About 80,000 blocks in 65 communities heavily infested with rats applied these criteria in their IPM efforts and attained an essentially rat-free and environmentally improved status. Hence, this set of criteria became widely accepted as the tolerance limit for a block, target area, or community. Local rodent IPM authorities may establish tolerance limits for other deficiency categories as needed. Tolerance limits will provide evaluative feedback to determine the direction to be taken by a rodent IPM program.

Table 2. Types of Major Exterior Deficiencies and Associated Colors on a GIS Map		
Categories	**Premises Deficient (%)***	**Color on Map**
Rodent Infestation		
Active Rodent Signs	None in block	Blue
	2% or less	Green
	2%–25%	Yellow
	26%–100%	Red
Rodent Food		
Unapproved Refuse Storage	None in block	Blue
	30% or less	Green
	30%–60%	Yellow
	61%–100%	Red
Exposed Garbage	None in block	Blue
	15% or less	Green
	15%–30%	Yellow
	31%–100%	Red

*Percentages have been rounded to the nearest whole number.

Infestation is calculated as the number of premises with active rodent signs divided by the total number of premises on a block times 100.

Comprehensive surveys (i.e., premises-by-premises) to identify active rodent signs and their causative conditions should be conducted, at a minimum, twice yearly for all blocks that have not reached the tolerance limits for active rodent signs, exposed garbage, or unapproved refuse storage. Comprehensive inspections should continue until 80% or more of the blocks in a target area have achieved the established tolerance limit and have maintained that status for at least 1 year. Thereafter, a sample survey procedure may be used two or more times a year to verify the status of the target area blocks that have achieved the tolerance limit; for the other blocks, comprehensive inspections should be conducted at least twice yearly.

If the survey data indicate that conditions have deteriorated and that rates of active rodent signs, exposed garbage, and unapproved refuse storage have risen above the tolerance limit, appropriate IPM interventions will be required based on the analysis of the data.

Interior Tolerance Limits

Interior inspections require visiting every room of every unit or every location of a structure on a premises. These visits provide inspectors with a detailed profile of the infestation and its causative conditions. One difficulty in this aspect of an urban IPM program is that inspectors are not likely to gain entry to all premises, units, or locations.

From the standpoint of good public health practice, the tolerance limit for rats or mice in human living quarters should be zero; that is, rodents should not live with people. To achieve and sustain a zero-tolerance limit for rodent infestation for one or more dwelling units, the same criteria should apply as that for exterior exposed garbage and unapproved refuse storage.

For interior surveys, the following additional broad-scale tolerance limit should be established:

15% or less of the premises with rodent entry and access routes within 5 feet (1.5 meters) of grade or other low horizontal surfaces.

This tolerance limit for entry and access routes may not fully address the problem of rodent access to exterior premises, but it greatly increases the likelihood of achieving the zero tolerance limit for rodents in dwelling units, a key quality-of-life issue. This limit also promotes the application of rodent-stoppage interventions that are essential to reducing interior infestation.

•••••••••

The urban rodent survey is an essential tool in the IPM effort to manage rodent problems. The survey provides precise information about infestations and their causative conditions, and it measures progress toward their elimination.

This manual should serve as a basis for designing and conducting valid surveys to determine the magnitude of infestation problems and their causes, for implementing interventions, and for measuring progress. The survey, however, is only a framework for the many activities of a rodent IPM program. An IPM program cannot succeed without the commitment of the local health authority, other professionals, and the public.

•••••••••

Selected References

Center for Disease Control. National urban rat control project directors meeting; 1974 Apr 30–May 2; Atlanta, Georgia. Atlanta: US Department of Health, Education, and Welfare; 1974.

Center for Disease Control. Urban rat surveys. Atlanta: US Department of Health, Education, and Welfare; 1974.

Center for Disease Control. Urban rat control program survey methodology. Atlanta: US Department of Health, Education, and Welfare; 1975.

Center for Disease Control. Urban rat control program: interior rat control: definitions and criteria. Atlanta: US Department of Health, Education, and Welfare; 1977.

Center for Disease Control. Urban rat control program: roof rat control: definitions and criteria. Atlanta: US Department of Health, Education, and Welfare; 1977.

Centers for Disease Control. Urban rat surveys. Atlanta: US Department of Health and Human Services; 1980. HHS publication number CDC 80-8344.

Davis DE. In: Houk VN, editor. Focus: urban rat control/environmental health abstracts. Atlanta: US Department of Health, Education, and Welfare; 1976.

Frantz SC. Evaluation of rodent infestations in Nepal: a preliminary report. J Nepal Med Assoc. 1974:12(3–4):17–32.

Frantz SC. The behavioral/ecological milieu of godown bandicoot rats—implications for environmental manipulation. In: Proceedings of the All India Rodent Seminar, Ahmedabad, Rodent Control Project; 1975 Sep 23–26, Sidhpur, Gujarat, India. Sidhpur, Gujarat, India: Rodent Control Project; 1977. p. 95–101.

Frantz SC. Rodent control: a case for integrated pest management program (IPM). In: Preventive Health Services Conference; 1979 May 7–11; Ellenville, New York. Atlanta: US Department of Health, Education, and Welfare; 1979.

Frantz SC. Architecture and commensal vertebrate pest management. In: Kundsin RB, editor. Architectural design and indoor microbial pollution. New York: Oxford University Press; 1988. p. 228–95.

Frantz SC. Integrated pest management in New York State. IPM Practitioner. 1996;18(2):8–10.

Frantz SC, Comings JP. 1976. Evaluation of urban rodent infestations—An approach in Nepal. In: Siebe CC, editor. Proceedings of the Seventh Vertebrate Pest Conference; 1976 Mar 9–11; Monterey, California. Davis, CA: University of California at Davis. p. 279–90.

Frantz SC, Davis DE. Bionomics and integrated pest management of commensal rodents. In: Gorham JR, editor. Ecology and management of food-industry pests. FDA Technical Bulletin 4. Arlington, VA: Association of Official Analytical Chemists. 1991. p. 243–313.

Frantz SC, Gallagher D. IPM implementation in New York State government facilities. In: Seventeenth Vertebrate Pest Conference; 1996 Mar 4–7.Rohnert Park, CA. Davis, CA: University of California at Davis. 1996.

Littig KS, Bjornson BF, Pratt HD, Fehn CF. Urban rat surveys. Washington, DC: US Department of Health, Education, and Welfare; no date. Available at URL: http://courses.washington.edu/envh442/Readings/Reading03.pdf.

Centers for Disease Control and Prevention, National Center for Environmental Health. Managing rodents and mosquitoes through integrated pest management [video]. A Public Health Training Network Satellite Broadcast, 2003 Sep 18. Atlanta: US Department of Health and Human Services; 2003.

Appendix A—Survey Forms

Figure 1. Block Record—Exterior Rodent Inspection and Sanitation Form (blank)

BLOCK RECORD—EXTERIOR RODENT INSPECTION AND SANITATION FORM

City: _____ County: _____

Census Tract: _____ Block Number: _____

Inspector(s): _____ Inspector(s) Initials: _____

Additional Block Information: _____

Date: ___ mm dd yy

Page: ___ of ___ Pages

No.	Premises Address	Premises Type				Premises Details				Food				Water			Harborage								Entry/Access			
		1. Residential	2. Commercial & Residential	3. Commercial	4. Vacant Lot	5. Food-Commercial	6. Vacant	7. No. of Dwelling Units	8. Sewers on Premises	9. Unapproved Refuse Storage	10. Exposed Garbage	11. Animal Food	12. Other Food & Plants	13. Standing Water	14. Condensate	15. Leaks	16. Abandoned Vehicles	17. Abandoned Appliances	18. Lumber/Clutter on Ground	19. Other Large Rubbish	20. Outbuildings/Privies	21. Board Fences & Walls	22. Plant-Related	23. Structural Deficiencies	24. Pipe/Wiring Gaps	25. Active Signs
	TOTAL																										

Remarks (continue on back of form as necessary):

Figure 2. Block Record—Exterior Rodent Inspection and Sanitation Form (completed example)

BLOCK RECORD—EXTERIOR RODENT INSPECTION AND SANITATION FORM

City: Metropolis
County: Chandler

Census Tract: 54-A
Block Number: 27

Inspector(s): H. Smith, A. Jones
Initials: HS, AJ

Additional Block Information: 15 premises total accessed

Date: 07 (mm) 26 (dd) 05 (yy)
Page 1 **of** 2 **Pages**

Block map: Ruskin St (top), King Ave, Chavez Ave, Biko St; N (arrow pointing left/west)

Column groupings — Premises Type (1–4), Premises Details (5–8), Food (9–12), Water (13–15), Harborage (16–22), Entry/Access (23–25)

No.	Premises Address	1. Residential	2. Commercial & Residential	3. Commercial	4. Vacant Lot	5. Food-Commercial	6. Vacant	7. No. of Dwelling Units	8. Sewers on Premises	9. Unapproved Refuse Storage	10. Exposed Garbage	11. Animal Food	12. Other Food & Plants	13. Standing Water	14. Condensate	15. Leaks	16. Abandoned Vehicles	17. Abandoned Appliances	18. Lumber/Clutter on Ground	19. Other Large Rubbish	20. Outbuildings/Privies	21. Board Fences & Walls	22. Plant-Related	23. Structural Deficiencies	24. Pipe/Wiring Gaps	25. Active Signs
1	646 Ruskin St.	✓						6	✓	✓	✓					✓					✓		✓	✓		✓
2	648 Ruskin St.	✓						4		✓	✓	✓	✓									✓		✓		
3	650 Ruskin St.				✓			0										✓	✓	✓					✓	✓
4	652 Ruskin St.	✓						8		✓	✓	✓											✓			✓
5	654 Ruskin St.	✓						6		✓												✓		✓		
6	[Chavez Ave.; data not shown]	—	—	—	—	—	—	—	—	—	—	—	—	—	—	—	—	—	—	—	—	—	—	—	—	—
7	661 Biko St.	✓						4		✓	✓		✓	✓		✓					✓					✓
8	663 Biko St.	✓						3		✓	✓			✓										✓		
9	[King St; data not shown]	—	—	—	—	—	—	—	—	—	—	—	—	—	—	—	—	—	—	—	—	—	—	—	—	—
10	1243 King St.	✓						2		✓	✓											✓				✓
	TOTAL	7	0	0	1	0	0	33	1	7	6	2	2	2	0	2	0	1	1	1	2	3	2	4	1	5

Remarks (continue on back of form as necessary):

Figure 3. Summary—Exterior Rodent Inspection and Sanitation Form (blank)

SUMMARY—EXTERIOR RODENT INSPECTION AND SANITATION FORM

Number of Premises With Deficiencies

| City: | | County: | Census Tract: | Block Number: | Inspector(s): | Inspector(s) Initials: | Additional Information: | Date | Page | of | Pages | mm | dd | yy |

Premises Type					Premises Details						Food				Water			Harborage							Entry/Access			
1. Residential	2. Commercial & Residential	3. Commercial	4. Vacant Lot	5. Food-Commercial	6. Vacant	7. No of Dwelling Units	8. Sewers on Premises	9. Unapproved Refuse Storage	10. Exposed Garbage	11. Animal Food	12. Other Food & Plants	13. Standing Water	14. Condensate	15. Leaks	16. Abandoned Vehicles	17. Abandoned Appliances	18. Lumber/Clutter on Ground	19. Other Large Rubbish	20. Outbuildings/Privies	21. Board Fences & Walls	22. Plant-Related	23. Structural Deficiencies	24. Pipe/Wiring Gaps	25. Active Signs

Number of Premises

Block Number

Total

Percent

Remarks (continue on back of form as necessary):

Figure 4. Summary—Exterior Rodent Inspection and Sanitation Form (completed example)

SUMMARY—EXTERIOR RODENT INSPECTION AND SANITATION FORM
Number of Premises With Deficiencies

City: Metropolis
County: Chandler
Census Tract: 54-A
Block Number: 27
Inspector(s): H. Smith, A. Jones
Inspector(s): Initials: HS, AJ
Additional Information:
Date: 07 / 26 / 05 (mm/dd/yy)
Page 1 of 1 — Pages 1

Block Number	Number of Premises	1. Residential	2. Commercial & Residential	3. Commercial	4. Vacant Lot	5. Food-Commercial	6. Vacant	7. No of Dwelling Units	8. Sewers on Premises	9. Unapproved Refuse Storage	10. Exposed Garbage	11. Animal Food	12. Other Food & Plants	13. Standing Water	14. Condensate	15. Leaks	16. Abandoned Vehicles	17. Abandoned Appliances	18. Lumber/Clutter on Ground	19. Other Large Rubbish	20. Outbuildings/Privies	21. Board Fences & Walls	22. Plant-Related	23. Structural Deficiencies	24. Pipe/Wiring Gaps	25. Active Signs
				Premises Type				Premises Details		Food				Water			Harborage							Entry/Access		
27	15	10	2	2	1	2	2	38	2	11	8	5	2	3	1	1	2	1	1	4	0	5	5	8	3	6
28	15	6	3	6	0	2	0	20	0	9	7	2	3	3	0	0	1	1	0	4	0	2	4	9	5	4
29	9	9	0	0	0	0	0	36	2	6	6	0	0	0	0	0	2	1	0	3	0	2	2	4	2	3
30	22	22	0	0	2	0	4	30	2	12	8	3	2	4	2	0	1	1	3	6	0	0	6	5	6	7
Total	220	195	4	7	14	4	22	264	18	115	85	12	12	21	6	9	8	12	10	38	4	18	30	70	14	50
Percent		89	2	3	6	2	10	NA	8	52	39	6	6	10	3	4	4	6	5	17	2	8	14	32	6	23

Remarks (continue on back of form as necessary):

Appendix B—Selecting a Random Sample

Suppose there is a finite population from which we wish to draw random sample of N elements. One method of creating a random sample would be to assign a number to each number of the population (e.g., block), put a set of numbered tags corresponding to the elements into a box, shake the box, and draw N tags from it. The numbers on these N tags would correspond to the elements to be selected. This method could be satisfactory, but it would require considerable labor to prepare the tags.

Instead of preparing numbered tags, we can use a table of random numbers. Such a table consists of numbers chosen in a fashion similar to drawing numbered tags out of a box. The table is so created that all numbers 0, 1... 9 appear with approxi¬mately the same frequency. By combining numbers in pairs, we have numbers from 00 to 99; by combining the numbers three at a time we have numbers from 000 to 999. The numbers can be combined as much as necessary.

Table B-1 is a table of random numbers that can be used to select a random sample. The starting point in the table should be selected randomly; one method is to close your eyes and place your finger on a page of the table.

Example

To select at random 20 blocks from a total population of 427 blocks in the area to be surveyed, assign the numbers 1 through 427 to the 427 blocks. To assign these numbers, use a map of the area so that each block is clearly defined.

Because 427 is a three digit number, combine three columns in the table and read them together. (For a two-digit number, combine and read two columns; for a four-digit number, combine and read four columns.) A column is a single-digit list of vertical numbers. In this table, columns are grouped in pairs.

- Select a starting point on the table randomly.

- If the number at the starting point is 427 or less, select the block having that number.

- If the number of the starting point is greater, continue down the horizontal rows until the number 427 or less is reached, and select that number.

- In either case, continue down the rows and, if necessary, down the columns beginning at the top of the page until 20 numbers of 427 or less have been located.

- This list will be the 20 blocks surveyed.

NOTES: Ignore any number over 427 because only 427 blocks exist in the total population to be surveyed. Having the same number 427 or less more than once does not matter. Continue until 20 numbers are selected.

Assuming 20 blocks will be chosen from a total population of 427 blocks, the selection process can be illustrated as follows:

- Suppose the randomly chosen starting point is the number formed by vertical columns 25–27 (remember that each digit is a column) in the 28th horizontal row of the third page of random numbers (page B-4).

- This number is **724**, which is more than 427, so continue down the same columns by horizontal row until the number **081** is reached. Block 81 would be the first block chosen.

The other 19 blocks chosen would be **361**, **373**, **61** (ignore 533 because it is over 427), **164**, **224**, **118** (ignore 876 and 948), **300**, **9** (ignore 565 and 613), **140** (ignore 724, 453, and 717), **38** (move to the top of the page, vertical columns 28–30 for the remaining numbers) **401**, **225**, **233**, **328**, **5**, **184**, **117**, **376**, and **114**.

- The last nine blocks chosen (beginning with **401**) are found in the numbers formed by combining columns 28–30 in row 1 on the same page.

Table B-1. Random Numbers Table

60	06	47	98	21	58	56	49	01	56	73	29	70	96	79	51	75	51	54	10	04
51	81	17	58	66	30	25	87	71	58	60	02	14	93	62	47	90	05	72	42	66
11	18	29	73	19	41	31	89	19	46	89	30	16	01	67	24	05	63	84	66	08
58	88	55	05	34	64	70	94	96	64	64	82	20	70	86	81	05	47	94	85	92
39	67	26	49	19	64	88	49	12	25	36	06	64	90	10	52	82	07	81	00	44
32	28	93	65	47	82	15	40	03	55	25	77	89	24	12	80	25	89	26	72	34
73	07	31	96	78	95	93	63	77	81	19	84	56	57	98	26	49	00	91	25	97
55	38	86	81	02	24	41	55	37	14	04	63	99	10	03	94	94	77	94	91	30
42	93	75	26	51	78	95	91	26	47	84	53	38	77	77	90	05	46	79	57	93
60	01	06	66	01	73	18	11	12	99	17	36	06	48	49	07	62	67	25	36	21
94	86	84	71	72	48	27	15	89	10	58	67	24	18	19	51	67	18	26	94	77
77	89	23	86	79	60	02	64	79	64	81	16	15	88	44	37	50	48	56	48	67
17	85	77	85	82	16	15	19	22	24	25	70	99	19	89	19	93	64	91	12	11
08	40	03	74	16	36	34	81	09	18	69	85	82	20	02	96	71	75	38	76	52
95	92	43	47	99	06	63	94	82	03	94	90	05	84	61	37	18	09	74	10	91
23	56	49	22	28	86	84	56	54	14	78	88	52	74	08	57	96	64	79	61	29
66	26	77	78	85	79	54	10	73	26	40	16	27	20	30	30	00	46	74	13	24
00	04	60	06	59	42	96	77	99	02	90	05	25	69	65	44	31	71	67	06	12
53	35	83	32	40	10	54	24	30	00	52	93	63	99	07	20	12	71	59	36	21
71	61	23	67	26	84	71	58	58	82	25	56	46	77	80	22	34	96	73	29	70
91	24	03	42	79	56	72	35	49	12	89	14	81	04	42	73	07	39	35	77	96
61	19	94	86	88	42	89	17	42	67	20	27	19	75	26	24	31	97	56	43	69
75	44	15	80	32	39	40	10	06	45	19	29	68	34	89	32	21	88	34	45	05
94	92	41	30	09	66	30	13	17	77	81	01	66	19	35	75	48	38	72	45	41
45	36	02	28	97	60	03	86	99	12	13	10	66	24	37	48	39	67	03	95	97
43	77	91	25	85	85	78	87	58	59	21	29	73	19	76	72	50	21	37	53	34
62	75	41	61	15	20	18	15	31	90	01	57	96	75	47	82	16	36	17	62	53
38	93	56	59	49	04	14	41	26	92	37	58	81	12	30	33	30	19	72	42	98
28	78	75	38	75	49	21	88	45	23	62	51	86	87	69	78	87	56	47	73	17
91	19	57	82	14	78	83	27	23	98	22	26	80	36	00	86	81	00	49	01	91
29	59	37	43	62	63	88	38	97	42	90	04	98	38	82	21	85	82	19	89	22
44	30	03	09	34	80	38	95	82	07	45	44	13	61	23	99	06	78	78	90	11
51	82	12	35	93	62	68	40	20	73	04	19	82	14	70	91	25	48	61	33	18
28	91	22	07	75	46	52	87	71	81	09	46	55	17	35	70	88	49	11	63	97
48	37	22	23	69	64	76	70	92	51	55	35	98	25	53	47	78	83	41	42	90
03	62	73	15	92	37	29	74	20	14	17	97	45	25	64	88	50	16	20	78	86
99	11	15	24	38	80	29	50	14	70	96	76	61	26	73	22	17	57	86	78	80
44	13	41	42	91	25	42	79	65	53	36	21	66	22	34	64	72	55	04	00	70
88	36	14	85	76	72	42	80	40	07	49	16	28	81	18	12	24	04	69	65	31
60	15	83	45	32	39	76	76	74	15	63	87	56	57	99	04	68	43	71	78	72
32	61	39	79	57	89	14	70	98	29	20	07	67	03	95	93	72	44	19	79	53
53	66	02	46	62	54	23	81	02	56	74	04	74	23	74	19	83	36	28	85	86
88	47	96	81	16	48	43	81	09	11	67	00	82	20	77	95	99	13	62	45	20
26	83	44	25	39	53	68	35	76	62	58	64	87	65	37	31	87	59	32	40	08
88	41	53	33	08	98	29	19	72	35	86	86	98	23	99	16	47	90	05	64	79
59	23	68	53	43	52	98	34	46	57	93	62	64	74	03	82	12	43	76	68	42
89	17	72	35	47	75	49	09	16	53	64	85	96	68	34	75	43	79	60	04	29
35	82	07	56	68	48	35	68	31	97	58	75	29	34	94	91	24	08	82	12	93

Table B-1. Random Numbers Table

87	69	76	54	25	83	30	47	87	68	31	63	95	85	81	09	02	52	99	18	14
85	86	90	10	02	23	92	43	61	33	04	35	58	58	80	25	73	16	13	42	99
17	81	10	27	04	24	25	89	23	88	49	08	82	10	95	99	13	66	21	74	05
90	05	48	61	28	81	07	46	75	44	32	78	96	74	00	23	84	62	73	19	96
76	53	45	31	94	96	69	74	02	44	32	34	63	80	30	22	22	43	58	67	13
09	12	33	32	61	25	93	71	71	70	94	81	00	74	24	24	15	78	71	58	56
68	51	69	71	71	73	09	95	99	17	88	53	47	78	79	53	57	99	07	62	64
87	69	61	40	02	37	38	84	68	53	33	10	75	40	01	38	94	85	75	40	16
17	54	28	83	50	48	62	68	54	00	40	14	35	53	36	33	10	90	09	33	19
61	12	25	56	64	90	10	55	08	20	19	67	04	05	73	05	85	90	02	94	94
91	27	01	70	90	10	07	29	29	68	34	77	78	81	18	01	52	88	39	55	20
08	68	36	23	79	50	17	49	01	85	91	17	86	96	78	91	28	75	35	79	49
11	01	37	34	81	06	35	55	18	41	63	98	23	84	60	02	10	25	59	54	25
62	45	43	61	15	58	76	60	07	45	11	73	06	59	48	53	68	42	81	21	99
07	72	52	90	07	74	11	85	83	45	18	23	95	85	79	68	40	15	49	04	67
09	81	06	78	94	90	08	90	02	52	85	84	68	57	96	64	64	89	26	57	90
05	28	71	66	12	10	70	93	69	65	48	54	09	52	78	92	37	63	83	48	58
58	76	74	06	32	38	95	86	92	39	65	45	03	88	34	45	15	48	35	84	65
51	68	40	03	11	63	99	14	87	57	98	25	52	74	23	97	53	41	28	96	76
70	87	69	76	53	44	03	25	93	60	18	16	11	98	25	71	63	93	56	42	96
79	51	61	13	09	47	94	78	73	10	33	01	49	00	00	88	46	50	29	35	78
84	65	49	12	96	64	78	75	40	20	06	88	54	17	87	59	53	36	09	10	36
29	69	73	17	87	78	88	55	25	85	96	67	21	79	47	98	32	44	15	11	90
00	14	78	76	73	03	48	55	34	96	65	40	18	07	37	61	23	87	58	70	93
64	80	31	80	40	28	83	47	97	57	96	74	06	39	68	39	82	27	17	77	80
35	68	50	37	14	65	35	74	20	45	31	94	80	32	32	44	37	55	15	43	78
87	71	68	41	61	40	25	32	71	63	87	65	36	14	96	73	10	88	50	17	76
51	73	16	52	80	29	30	10	72	52	82	20	69	65	33	36	36	01	18	59	24
25	70	88	35	50	19	20	04	60	19	51	67	24	25	63	91	20	49	11	95	85
90	10	17	84	62	59	54	10	18	13	14	90	10	57	91	17	47	89	12	92	42
82	14	58	68	47	93	67	27	39	56	45	14	96	70	92	37	46	78	75	35	49
09	41	40	05	33	19	74	20	09	31	73	09	86	86	88	53	65	47	72	38	96
66	14	86	97	58	78	85	85	98	36	31	98	28	83	44	41	61	28	93	58	75
39	36	34	64	87	58	67	12	02	01	95	96	77	85	89	22	51	75	30	08	87
77	87	75	26	53	59	37	15	99	02	81	10	54	16	37	41	27	48	42	90	10
64	92	33	27	40	00	33	12	52	95	93	59	44	41	46	62	60	04	26	33	18
69	79	53	44	24	06	94	83	30	47	87	65	42	80	30	04	03	52	98	26	59
24	03	07	16	12	85	96	80	27	52	97	45	15	73	24	14	93	70	89	22	45
38	84	62	59	38	70	90	01	62	69	80	30	21	54	28	84	61	38	90	10	67
16	14	60	06	47	80	25	68	53	35	97	51	62	47	98	39	37	34	80	22	07
88	53	37	15	16	23	73	14	84	55	26	78	90	01	36	01	69	84	60	17	32
43	42	92	46	63	92	38	89	25	87	55	32	19	37	44	00	75	26	22	16	29
39	65	54	12	90	01	86	82	07	01	92	45	19	74	20	60	17	29	24	11	74
22	10	52	93	59	48	33	22	06	95	97	59	40	06	92	41	36	38	85	78	84
55	08	09	91	16	62	73	19	92	37	23	63	86	97	56	74	00	88	33	01	82
08	32	37	57	97	58	73	26	89	19	29	13	24	41	60	20	56	58	88	41	56
69	73	13	05	16	08	89	13	00	37	19	54	03	34	96	79	65	56	57	97	48
32	73	13	20	17	94	89	31	90	01	84	53	46	88	53	46	57	98	23	77	97

84	55	38		87	70	94		82	10	44		19	35	45		16	14	01
27	17	56		60	16	17		73	07	33		37	57	91		11	82	25
30	53	36		31	81	08		81	06	76		53	66	07		11	68	41
12	21	90		07	82	03		16	28	76		73	07	62		44	35	69
96	73	07		90	10	87		71	82	17		56	69	81		20	72	33
76	66	10		40	07	95		89	18	16		23	77	87		56	48	42

05 90 06   17 39 80
72 38 95   88 38 91
56 59 49   07 25 44
77 97 47   93 57 77
36 15 56   70 98 28
97 56 48   29 16 55

05	16	12	73	25	48	27	19	49	09	11	91	15	83	28
30	36	12	40	17	56	54	29	15	70	89	15	68	36	31
27	05	29	12	27	32	50	28	99	05	88	42	95	90	05
05	14	71	77	91	27	01	73	12	24	08	80	37	28	90
25	62	57	97	56	60	12	95	94	90	05	28	93	67	01
19	60	10	44	34	65	47	68	44	20	70	88	48	55	35

58 65 33   08 58 59
84 62 56   49 08 24
35 82 12   32 39 49
08 54 12   17 55 36
88 39 75   35 76 60
45 06 44   26 19 75

33	12	13	69	65	32	41	23	86	95	89	15	82	21	84
71	62	70	87	66	21	83	41	47	84	67	10	65	36	30
63	84	61	35	49	04	59	39	38	97	50	22	50	39	45
21	74	01	30	44	28	90	05	92	54	25	50	52	99	01
88	35	82	23	87	65	35	81	13	28	75	35	50	37	57
58	62	44	36	09	68	34	91	27	42	91	29	67	07	69

62 61 15   99 09 51
07 68 37   54 04 07
14 06 26   50 27 18
73 17 87   59 46 86
98 26 51   67 24 18
83 42 98   38 99 15

76	69	68	41	18	27	38	80	41	23	97	60	14	91	17
79	61	39	79	51	70	93	66	08	44	02	08	17	63	76
06	92	53	46	77	93	67	13	24	25	85	94	78	94	93
86	96	68	41	19	69	72	45	06	08	83	50	33	16	05
78	72	45	15	68	52	94	96	73	09	49	20	23	81	14
10	90	06	81	04	68	40	17	99	06	55	08	35	64	63

78 78 84   65 61 11
67 16 38   96 77 81
68 47 90   08 44 34
31 84 72   39 38 96
23 72 44   08 03 73
87 60 07   98 24 26

93	58	71	67	19	82	23	72	51	85	80	30	21	86	94
31	78	77	97	51	65	33	21	91	12	22	09	09	21	92
63	90	02	16	33	35	54	06	33	09	33	15	15	71	57
47	96	70	91	19	79	65	49	02	89	19	28	72	49	08
57	92	46	60	06	37	37	20	39	64	71	78	76	69	63
16	44	11	01	28	82	09	11	94	90	09	13	08	17	47

76 64 81   03 10 01
37 41 45   23 67 23
99 16 51   81 18 27
82 05 15   99 14 29
99 13 41   51 60 08
91 18 12   12 80 28

60	19	88	45	17	76	52	98	38	96	63	98	36	11	07
03	48	66	28	96	77	99	00	11	89	25	61	37	30	21
82	21	61	30	45	04	32	59	21	57	98	24	06	11	44
28	91	20	11	03	34	94	85	85	74	24	04	53	33	28
35	68	37	27	01	05	73	02	25	84	53	37	16	41	29
17	89	23	83	50	27	01	72	52	87	73	14	22	47	68

03 38 98   32 58 67
54 19 22   54 17 85
04 13 15   12 75 27
69 78 74   21 99 06
28 74 08   09 35 89
41 47 79   53 38 84

61	40	15	89	20	66	13	07	43	79	68	40	11	84	57
44	20	21	47	79	48	64	71	78	83	28	86	87	67	23
10	20	06	68	35	64	63	90	06	14	76	57	94	89	31
08	86	97	40	06	15	77	78	93	71	71	72	30	04	08
36	14	78	74	17	99	16	21	74	01	55	14	00	96	73
26	80	36	02	17	80	39	38	67	00	08	87	56	54	18

82 26 27   31 87 56
88 51 86   85 87 60
92 37 17   43 74 18
47 83 50   41 58 88
23 56 69   83 38 91
76 55 22   02 39 61

22	27	01	34	56	48	32	61	40	21	38	87	61	37	49
96	80	34	42	87	60	03	99	16	25	55	08	14	04	04
44	29	20	03	62	69	71	71	69	84	67	23	72	42	97
74	08	31	79	67	24	16	05	35	43	58	88	45	39	53
01	86	95	83	38	65	36	08	24	17	67	26	71	73	18
08	29	63	76	55	17	88	51	72	51	90	03	03	86	83

16 56 58   79 59 38
16 36 07   91 18 16
46 54 23   60 02 71
57 93 63   90 02 66
67 00 88   45 19 99
49 17 92   45 37 63

Table B-1. Random Numbers Table

09	93	60	20	52	82	14	15	13	38	92	50	36	35	47	81	01	96	85	45	15
76	59	42	82	10	80	32	37	11	90	00	10	43	87	65	33	02	52	94	82	12
00	95	97	52	94	86	79	49	09	30	49	10	72	34	94	77	97	57	97	41	33
12	03	84	69	60	01	75	36	14	81	19	27	16	24	29	64	71	63	80	33	07
01	39	74	06	35	60	06	09	17	94	88	53	58	59	38	70	90	09	53	61	26
64	87	56	62	65	43	69	82	06	87	67	08	90	06	62	68	43	65	34	71	66
12	94	88	42	95	90	07	60	17	96	63	99	07	89	19	62	56	50	50	38	95
92	45	35	52	93	74	07	35	89	13	20	34	98	36	17	75	28	94	91	16	47
86	84	62	63	79	69	83	29	53	34	92	40	13	21	76	69	71	71	69	86	97
54	01	30	02	32	63	79	46	89	29	36	22	27	15	85	90	08	48	57	96	79
58	81	12	61	27	40	19	89	30	36	43	87	60	80	20	08	38	93	68	50	27
13	61	33	03	17	43	73	06	53	56	45	46	54	10	89	28	88	34	50	18	26
93	74	19	47	91	13	43	49	05	87	71	83	45	32	71	61	17	33	12	33	14
72	40	09	56	42	68	57	94	79	56	68	32	34	87	64	64	65	39	68	45	36
09	61	25	90	03	72	55	32	31	83	36	09	45	13	27	41	53	59	39	40	05
70	94	79	61	43	54	12	95	92	50	50	27	02	98	36	39	71	69	83	31	59
49	23	70	87	75	29	26	30	47	98	22	48	42	77	99	09	65	40	07	84	67
21	89	12	02	56	41	58	70	94	90	07	39	63	87	69	85	96	67	21	67	25
56	45	23	67	25	84	55	17	90	02	24	46	73	08	28	59	28	90	04	99	03
67	19	98	33	30	47	98	33	02	48	59	47	70	93	70	99	09	26	68	30	28
76	76	77	79	71	83	33	39	40	07	73	05	91	18	11	50	36	20	19	43	67
07	01	28	58	59	53	60	19	58	85	82	15	09	02	15	71	72	34	77	88	46
78	87	66	28	78	90	07	44	03	62	52	94	88	50	52	94	91	21	79	61	20
38	83	38	68	34	49	03	34	73	18	22	25	68	47	99	13	61	18	17	47	49
22	02	68	34	87	72	34	79	57	75	48	29	26	29	62	73	15	35	68	51	79
50	38	91	20	34	70	96	64	64	85	76	53	67	24	21	73	22	52	84	64	62
51	84	53	55	34	49	05	23	92	45	07	83	34	63	97	42	90	03	35	46	49
04	83	41	46	61	42	86	78	79	64	65	34	85	97	47	84	52	84	67	18	18
66	31	58	71	80	31	95	92	50	22	59	43	50	38	66	27	47	96	73	07	11
40	08	17	85	88	33	01	63	78	80	38	76	56	75	25	92	39	58	84	54	06
14	11	47	92	47	93	73	03	12	51	59	49	01	63	86	91	13	03	64	82	11
66	06	95	84	57	93	67	05	68	44	27	36	04	45	03	75	39	48	37	55	32
60	04	39	40	01	67	16	21	37	61	30	20	74	22	28	86	98	24	09	94	77
94	95	97	48	34	43	75	39	57	96	68	35	80	38	65	60	16	02	08	11	80
33	16	28	79	52	99	08	34	43	56	75	41	51	83	28	93	66	02	09	30	42
44	05	05	84	59	31	59	32	46	49	07	22	43	80	38	86	91	32	90	04	
13	10	55	40	20	56	43	78	87	60	07	17	30	05	22	15	59	26	73	09	12
51	87	62	62	49	22	42	84	64	68	38	98	24	44	00	67	00	40	12	59	44
13	64	89	23	99	04	48	27	40	21	97	55	22	60	12	43	84	60	03	10	62
53	67	17	92	46	62	61	23	54	01	95	96	68	47	95	98	36	00	66	11	53
54	00	28	87	58	70	97	51	81	18	27	33	10	48	27	49	01	92	51	53	46
64	84	61	43	73	21	99	19	53	64	80	42	68	51	65	35	62	74	17	35	47
83	37	33	08	57	89	22	01	38	77	83	45	39	48	62	46	74	05	91	13	62
47	90	01	85	81	17	63	96	67	16	05	40	14	74	19	27	00	45	46	87	70
91	24	07	68	56	47	68	54	01	88	42	88	49	06	98	38	93	68	51	80	38
96	64	66	03	55	20	36	16	47	90	01	76	75	50	42	89	26	73	24	00	19
25	50	48	39	60	07	92	38	85	79	70	90	06	85	83	29	53	41	61	12	71
70	94	87	59	24	03	33	15	84	51	71	59	25	76	76	53	46	86	99	05	52

95	97	43	49	15	65	41	28	73	09	13	22	04	17	31	77	93	71	61	30	38
79	61	20	28	58	58	86	99	06	53	40	14	61	26	25	93	68	35	80	42	99
17	87	63	85	75	24	21	89	19	71	80	40	09	50	39	79	55	10	90	03	09
70	97	53	41	43	47	68	47	90	08	35	71	73	16	04	28	80	31	70	89	14
01	72	48	55	25	32	69	63	92	53	37	53	59	41	45	42	73	23	70	96	69
70	92	39	50	46	63	92	38	72	54	13	36	19	95	84	67	06	09	21	69	59
34	93	61	16	63	80	43	81	02	48	30	12	29	31	99	10	38	73	13	23	73
21	90	06	24	09	50	43	63	80	33	15	53	34	92	41	60	02	38	97	51	83
30	25	96	63	94	94	96	79	59	48	67	04	73	18	15	94	88	53	38	67	21
61	11	58	59	52	96	64	87	66	09	90	00	91	19	62	75	34	83	29	60	00
64	73	04	84	70	90	02	28	86	87	75	36	16	32	47	76	64	78	93	73	05
73	13	52	98	22	19	88	49	18	42	79	57	95	97	59	29	24	26	92	53	47
92	52	89	14	56	60	17	56	48	32	30	31	63	77	77	90	09	84	69	69	81
15	78	96	78	84	52	99	18	29	40	10	40	28	59	42	84	70	97	44	32	32
19	91	31	62	51	85	85	76	57	99	09	54	15	60	13	11	02	99	15	35	82
16	61	40	02	31	89	26	44	09	01	94	92	50	17	72	55	35	65	34	68	33
06	30	02	96	74	07	60	09	79	51	81	10	03	55	26	45	39	42	88	53	44
32	60	07	67	06	26	82	07	62	65	43	44	06	12	33	28	56	50	19	44	07
99	11	07	15	07	96	66	15	94	81	20	49	10	40	10	70	97	42	68	43	50
31	61	35	73	13	60	09	86	94	94	80	27	52	84	59	44	13	24	00	35	80
41	28	83	45	44	00	64	79	53	36	31	65	45	23	82	08	57	94	90	00	28
96	65	44	19	26	67	13	28	94	76	58	55	19	97	40	13	09	58	83	32	39
35	47	69	66	15	87	61	21	36	01	77	90	06	61	16	00	85	78	94	84	60
06	96	69	66	20	04	71	71	73	08	55	10	18	51	55	32	20	53	62	66	17
93	68	39	35	69	66	23	72	44	02	71	75	42	93	72	32	70	91	11	78	92
52	91	30	13	29	42	96	72	34	84	56	50	39	71	67	21	50	25	56	74	11
40	16	08	75	45	04	70	90	09	20	52	94	88	41	23	65	54	03	62	46	51
72	30	04	83	45	03	28	81	20	18	01	14	26	51	73	21	52	79	55	27	18
20	46	76	73	21	77	82	08	44	06	50	47	86	96	80	38	92	35	99	12	07
73	17	63	95	98	22	03	07	80	39	52	71	60	06	39	72	38	90	08	03	38
65	48	46	77	90	10	23	60	14	16	01	87	72	48	54	16	58	64	81	02	18
15	91	29	59	32	19	95	83	29	29	14	89	24	08	61	32	32	70	96	76	65
37	60	00	15	91	30	55	23	72	56	71	63	94	90	08	99	03	51	83	29	70
97	43	63	89	19	76	67	21	53	61	20	28	58	60	12	53	40	07	92	37	43
64	87	78	88	54	00	83	35	82	13	53	49	07	76	67	16	04	06	80	24	50
48	58	85	80	38	80	23	62	63	99	02	56	70	96	81	18	26	91	18	12	02
16	09	21	93	76	55	27	18	20	03	00	60	07	93	57	90	00	34	45	16	37
47	89	10	56	65	35	93	66	06	78	72	51	74	03	01	55	39	35	92	36	08
23	94	84	58	70	90	01	98	35	52	89	26	46	63	79	46	73	25	85	93	69
85	81	01	04	89	32	55	14	00	31	81	06	62	48	45	35	60	12	14	93	74
15	13	03	45	40	30	42	79	47	79	57	76	73	17	80	21	65	35	56	55	24
28	85	88	40	04	24	06	14	43	61	43	59	39	48	52	84	60	20	01	15	78
95	91	15	75	40	03	30	49	07	52	93	57	75	48	53	59	26	64	81	05	58
81	12	10	61	21	67	16	10	34	88	34	89	31	83	36	23	96	72	38	70	85
87	65	53	43	48	36	35	51	88	47	97	52	94	84	69	84	56	63	84	56	43
46	52	93	71	84	69	64	62	54	07	95	97	42	93	63	80	25	53	51	75	26
29	68	41	41	52	70	86	97	51	78	71	63	92	44	05	29	72	39	47	92	48
36	04	89	15	10	65	56	64	85	95	89	13	47	90	09	11	91	28	92	46	81

52	88	40	03	69	80	36	28	99	10	71	82	06	02	50	50	52	74	08	58	63
94	96	79	69	65	32	72	53	59	29	56	70	89	33	14	01	13	40	10	01	38
97	44	25	99	06	67	12	99	14	82	10	80	24	03	44	31	94	80	27	09	45
43	77	89	13	28	75	47	84	56	47	98	35	71	75	29	25	27	46	60	10	83
38	79	54	02	14	93	59	33	41	45	28	70	94	89	12	93	56	61	15	66	26
85	97	43	52	94	81	19	30	42	79	60	04	22	31	94	88	44	00	34	65	57
75	48	41	23	90	07	95	81	00	54	09	41	33	15	20	30	07	62	75	31	96
80	46	53	61	00	52	82	11	26	47	96	72	43	48	65	46	66	08	62	64	82
24	46	82	26	69	81	18	60	03	66	02	36	40	17	87	77	92	41	18	37	55
32	77	94	84	68	38	68	44	02	28	67	12	80	31	85	78	91	28	80	38	87
76	75	37	63	76	60	09	74	01	39	41	52	81	01	13	73	03	43	46	78	81
11	96	71	74	12	58	75	34	45	36	01	47	85	87	62	62	53	42	69	80	30
33	14	41	34	67	19	70	87	59	45	11	71	82	26	91	17	89	21	82	19	27
30	03	47	69	85	75	48	54	28	92	36	01	37	63	98	28	94	82	09	63	97
47	97	43	55	16	45	05	38	68	32	37	62	59	53	52	94	91	29	21	97	41
25	99	14	97	49	00	64	78	80	29	74	19	80	28	54	00	46	74	01	44	02
06	36	42	92	53	64	72	41	45	28	73	15	50	50	33	01	65	58	75	26	25
83	47	86	96	64	62	68	44	01	49	07	37	25	63	82	08	38	98	31	72	32
64	68	52	93	74	05	69	81	09	50	43	79	49	02	80	37	56	45	41	55	24
10	61	37	44	05	63	93	58	72	56	55	21	99	09	09	49	04	15	59	49	06
26	68	42	95	92	42	99	07	44	00	19	93	54	00	97	44	27	08	06	33	02
03	71	60	01	80	24	52	72	32	57	95	83	33	40	07	81	02	65	61	24	16
13	10	04	62	57	92	49	22	01	16	51	89	30	05	31	81	07	11	13	27	13
63	95	98	20	71	65	56	57	77	79	61	31	87	63	76	59	34	97	51	73	24
01	61	15	54	04	17	68	31	82	08	81	05	11	48	38	80	37	57	85	87	77
98	31	80	42	88	47	99	08	96	72	29	41	29	10	96	79	49	03	11	46	79
50	18	62	72	42	95	99	15	39	35	79	65	58	57	86	83	39	81	17	53	69
62	55	15	68	43	66	03	01	60	13	74	07	79	50	21	71	67	26	34	58	59
54	23	67	11	64	75	47	74	06	20	03	98	35	75	45	03	12	24	08	78	71
67	18	30	09	64	64	84	57	97	44	25	60	00	29	55	18	01	03	07	65	49
09	98	31	88	38	75	43	69	80	37	15	25	28	54	13	57	99	14	95	86	90
08	39	45	03	00	48	59	27	32	26	54	15	82	18	12	61	31	72	54	01	83
41	28	82	23	59	42	70	98	20	31	96	79	61	16	03	92	40	09	85	98	38
65	41	23	62	63	91	32	34	57	78	95	98	25	84	67	14	93	61	39	50	15
43	60	07	96	70	91	13	21	91	21	70	94	95	92	46	74	21	85	88	34	87
77	90	07	96	66	23	73	10	69	78	73	16	64	77	96	69	62	63	88	42	98
35	54	18	78	89	20	00	81	09	10	91	14	94	78	88	46	50	26	55	28	92
39	51	76	65	35	58	62	64	75	41	21	73	25	73	12	80	22	51	69	76	75
44	38	97	45	14	64	91	19	99	08	56	55	17	83	33	30	26	63	87	60	00
86	87	77	79	56	45	04	02	84	55	33	05	60	10	88	42	69	61	21	54	31
65	42	80	45	28	77	94	77	96	71	77	91	17	93	66	30	07	74	23	57	77
87	65	54	23	71	75	49	01	66	26	37	22	40	05	67	12	22	09	05	33	38
96	62	52	71	76	65	34	91	30	18	30	23	68	37	48	28	82	22	15	23	81
07	71	84	68	46	83	49	15	47	92	48	34	61	18	26	29	15	92	49	02	96
79	50	40	09	64	79	64	71	60	10	17	68	34	69	86	98	31	86	86	99	02
61	29	12	30	48	53	38	99	06	03	03	78	72	52	83	28	98	24	11	81	01
94	93	56	40	01	32	63	87	78	89	28	88	39	63	92	43	58	63	86	91	32
55	13	51	86	82	09	73	03	21	40	28	88	51	90	05	76	63	89	21	78	95

59	30	34	80	22	39	68	50	45	44	11	15	49	09	54	15	19	25	57	83	29
72	55	35	70	89	13	79	70	90	11	29	20	42	97	45	15	91	25	99	13	20
74	15	71	81	18	15	84	52	79	54	15	64	74	11	00	38	99	15	17	92	41
50	23	93	75	28	92	46	62	43	42	96	72	50	51	74	17	67	09	60	11	57
86	84	52	97	48	64	91	15	69	68	33	06	21	93	58	69	67	18	15	77	96
70	92	34	92	53	59	40	06	71	59	44	22	14	07	02	21	50	21	78	82	19
88	41	24	18	02	88	34	52	86	82	20	12	06	35	94	87	62	49	17	53	55
40	31	97	57	91	17	73	05	52	94	79	66	29	58	80	42	91	23	98	25	98
36	32	71	68	34	64	89	19	65	42	98	23	75	48	57	99	16	42	89	14	78
93	73	23	81	08	32	47	73	11	80	42	95	84	68	43	79	55	05	33	38	81
01	94	84	52	80	41	19	90	09	67	18	40	18	65	33	16	48	26	28	81	18
18	28	77	96	71	77	90	00	32	36	00	56	74	09	70	94	95	89	28	87	61
30	35	89	31	92	47	68	36	06	66	18	11	02	37	58	76	51	63	89	33	15
62	49	19	21	36	21	50	36	06	11	26	40	06	52	84	64	79	61	35	59	24
44	01	55	27	32	74	12	83	40	09	08	99	10	47	94	82	24	06	54	28	66
16	19	48	62	67	10	64	63	80	38	97	47	90	11	09	92	53	43	80	39	36
01	76	52	94	85	81	05	05	11	34	68	51	59	50	16	38	98	37	18	16	22
05	33	06	84	63	80	46	53	62	48	50	26	35	78	85	89	22	00	70	98	40
26	85	77	81	17	79	49	03	95	97	54	04	39	53	59	43	77	89	21	90	03
77	90	00	99	01	80	23	92	37	53	33	21	71	71	68	41	42	69	64	90	05
54	00	97	51	75	25	38	98	35	50	40	02	13	26	77	87	70	92	42	92	49
13	06	92	51	90	10	93	65	51	79	63	98	25	97	46	89	17	90	09	50	34
67	25	31	86	86	80	23	59	40	09	13	52	73	11	75	26	70	92	37	64	77
98	35	50	16	49	22	13	34	84	54	28	98	27	31	90	01	51	91	27	19	24
19	95	89	15	97	47	97	49	14	76	70	95	82	25	64	75	44	32	20	10	59
30	08	47	79	56	72	43	72	47	97	43	58	75	41	63	78	91	20	09	93	58
62	60	12	70	94	94	95	84	69	62	47	72	39	73	08	32	41	62	72	53	59
42	66	03	38	70	85	88	44	32	38	70	99	01	81	08	44	10	86	98	20	66
21	94	96	73	28	86	98	23	94	94	82	18	44	19	93	67	20	02	17	69	60
11	85	82	14	91	13	28	86	87	64	87	64	92	34	76	68	43	56	59	50	49
01	62	57	87	75	50	36	35	58	84	58	55	37	34	47	92	44	15	43	53	43
65	44	20	29	32	42	84	59	30	40	25	85	96	70	92	52	79	71	72	31	85
94	96	67	15	65	42	69	79	51	59	52	77	90	10	59	50	41	33	35	56	64
90	01	07	77	83	31	94	91	25	53	34	74	16	20	55	11	51	65	35	63	81
00	32	24	06	33	16	32	73	13	79	57	89	15	88	41	31	76	70	85	97	55
12	07	45	45	24	19	70	87	68	53	68	33	11	65	57	80	45	41	22	54	08
30	20	04	75	41	20	61	13	50	48	56	60	05	46	50	43	69	69	84	55	28
95	92	44	12	71	78	88	40	02	70	88	50	17	75	31	92	36	08	35	58	61
24	38	99	15	16	32	69	84	53	46	69	66	20	58	86	98	35	86	86	80	27
31	97	57	83	31	59	52	91	27	14	68	49	14	82	19	71	64	86	93	57	89
22	18	17	44	04	20	11	48	52	80	41	58	77	83	35	62	51	82	10	20	29
38	92	37	59	22	15	56	58	66	16	08	90	10	66	27	11	60	08	94	89	14
75	40	03	57	96	70	89	27	12	80	28	91	20	18	06	21	71	61	34	55	39
37	16	03	01	82	07	28	95	83	47	97	52	82	20	31	88	39	71	62	70	88
43	42	77	79	68	54	16	04	76	62	67	16	21	95	98	26	64	87	74	03	62
51	61	12	23	89	20	52	89	23	92	43	64	67	11	17	60	00	49	06	74	14
67	26	20	48	30	12	22	52	85	80	24	07	96	65	31	81	09	70	86	90	09
93	63	98	33	03	36	13	39	75	33	05	98	35	46	77	85	86	80	22	22	39